Susan Curtis has worked with natural medicines since 1979. She originally trained as a homœopath, and has since studied and used other forms of natural healing including herbs and essential oils. For several years, Susan practiced homœopathy professionally at a clinic of natural medicine in London, but recently she has committed herself to writing, and helping people to treat themselves using natural remedies. She is a co-author of *Neal's Yard Natural Remedies* and *Natural Healing for Women* and author of *Essential Oils*. Susan has two young children and lives in South London.

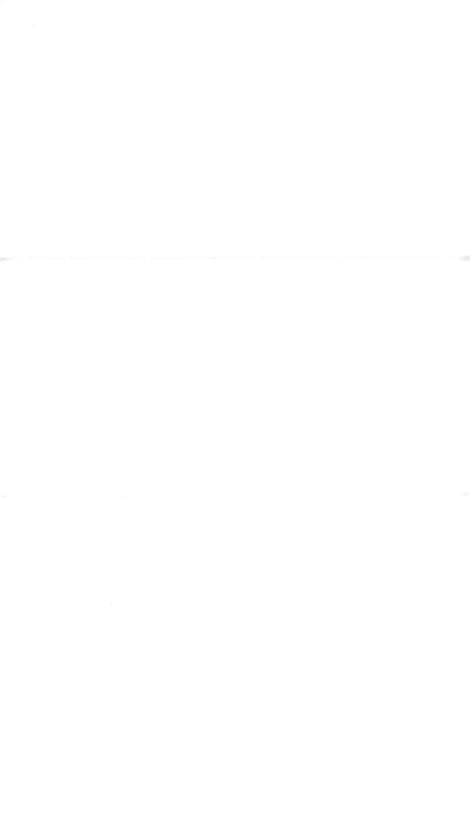

A Handbook
of
Homœopathic
Alternatives
to
Immunisation

Susan Curtis RSHom

Winter Press
16 Stambourne Way
West Wickham
Kent BR4 9NF

First published by Winter Press in 1994
Reprinted 1995, 1996
Revised 1999, Reprinted 2000

© Susan Curtis 1994

ISBN 1 874581 02 9

Cover design by David Loxley
Cover photo by Tony Boyce
Printed by Biddles of Guildford, Surrey

ACKNOWLEDGMENTS

With thanks to those homœopaths who willingly shared their experience; Kate Golding, Janice Micallef and Ernest Roberts. To Deborah Eastham and Sylvia Treacher for their valuable contributions. To Romy Fraser for her encouragement. To Gill Armstrong for editing the text. And to my husband, Colin Winter, for his help and support.

This book is presented as a collection of natural remedies and as an aid in understanding their use. It is not intended to replace or supersede professional consultation or treatment and no guarantee can be given as to the efficacy or appropriateness of a remedy in an individual case without professional advice.

CONTENTS

INTRODUCTION

As a homœopathic practitioner I was frequently asked what someone could do rather than be immunised when travelling abroad. In response I would write out a couple of pages of remedies and hand them over with an explanation of where to get them and how to take them. Many other homœopaths do the same, and several of them have mentioned how much they would like a book they could recommend to their patients that would contain practical advice.

There are several books available that detail the arguments against immunisation, (see the Suggested Reading section in the Appendices) and for this reason this book only briefly outlines the key issues, and concentrates rather on what individuals can do for themselves and their families having chosen to not be inoculated.

In 1986 I went to India for three months and had the opportunity to try out several of the remedies for myself. I did not have any inoculations. Other than a brief head cold as I adjusted to the formidable pollution of the Calcutta air, and a short but dramatic episode of food poisoning thanks to food being stored for three days at oven temperature in a ship's galley, I thoroughly enjoyed myself and stayed in good health.

I drank boiled water and took *Echinacea* tincture for a couple of weeks until I felt more confident about my body's ability to adjust to new conditions and took homœopathic remedies for the food poisoning and as a prophylactic for malaria during a boat trip along the Ganges. I was also very pleased to have access to a number of homœopathic suppliers in case I felt the need for any further remedies. Throughout India homœopathic remedies are widely available, in other areas of the world such as Africa and South America it will be necessary to take a reasonable stock of the most appropriate remedies with you.

Since having children I have been able to observe first hand the incredible vitality of an unvaccinated child. I have also come to understand the importance of parents having a basic knowledge of natural remedies so that they can step in at the early stages of a child's illness and prevent anything more frightening developing.

Many parents instinctively feel that pumping toxins into their children in the form of inoculations is wrong. It is the same process as dumping toxic waste into the rivers and oceans and expecting them to be healthy, life-supporting environments. As more and more parents choose not to immunise their children, so a knowledge of the alternative needs to become more widely available. This book has been written as a practical guide with this aim in mind.

Natural medicine has a great deal to offer both in the prevention and treatment of infectious diseases. I would encourage you to get a basic knowledge of the remedies, make contact with natural practitioners in your area and have confidence in your body's innate ability to heal itself when encouraged in the right direction.

PART I

CHAPTER I

THE CASE AGAINST IMMUNISATION

In 1993 the American Institute of Medicine report on vaccines concluded that virtually all the vaccines given to children have been proven to cause damage. Why is it that the medical profession has consistently underestimated the damage done by immunisations for so long, and why are they still being carried out?

Medical professionals recommend vaccines with the argument that immunisation has been responsible for the decline in infectious illnesses like diphtheria. In fact, because of better sanitation and hygiene, most of these diseases – such as diphtheria, cholera and typhoid – were in rapid and continuous decline well before the introduction of immunisation procedures.

Immunisation has been practiced for over a century and official reports have led us to believe that it has been responsible for the decline of infectious disease, and is effective in disease prevention. However, when the results have been re-examined using large sample groups, and taking into account other influencing factors, the claims for the effectiveness of immunisation appear to be unfounded and misleading.

A vaccine contains protein, bacterial and viral particles and also preservatives, neutralisers and carrying agents. It is an allergic reaction to these poisonous substances that causes the sudden collapse that can be very rapidly fatal known as anaphylactic shock. Immunisations for diphtheria, tetanus, hepatitis B, whooping cough and measles have all been found to cause cases of anaphylactic shock. Guillain-Barre syndrome, which causes paralysis, has been found to be caused by the immunisations for diphtheria, tetanus and the oral polio vaccine.

There is also mounting evidence for less immediate but equally devastating damage that is caused by vaccines. For example, the 1993 National Academy of Science Institute of Medicine (America) report found evidence that the rubella vaccine could cause short and long-term arthritis.

This longer term damage is a result of harm done to the immune system, particularly when done to the still developing immune system of a child. Viral elements injected into a child's body as vaccinations may persist and sometimes mutate in the system for years. It is now suggested that viral elements, such as those found in vaccines, can emerge later in the form of encephalitis, multiple sclerosis, rheumatoid arthritis and cancer.

Furthermore, as a result of injecting a vaccine directly into the body, only the antibody response is stimulated, as opposed to the normal process of illness and recovery. The inflammatory response to an infectious illness (for example, a fever, rash or cough) represents the body's natural efforts to clear the virus from the system. In this way the entire immune system is profoundly stimulated, and not only will the child who recovers from the illness have a natural immunity to it, but he will be able to respond rapidly and effectively to other infections. In fact, infectious diseases are necessary for the maturation of a healthy immune system, and this is particularly true of the common childhood illnesses such as chickenpox, measles and mumps.

So, why do doctors continue to immunise? Government statistics have consistently been manipulated to 'prove' the effectiveness of Government funded inoculation procedures. Research to 'prove' the effectiveness of individual inoculations has been funded by pharmaceutical companies who have a vested interest both in their sale, and also in playing down any possible damage they may cause. Orthodox medical schools have taught that inoculation is a benefit to the health of the nation without questioning whether or not this is true, and now many doctors are unwilling to face the consequences of throwing out such a massive part of their medical understanding. Furthermore, in the UK there are now financial incentives for doctors to encourage them to achieve immunisation targets. This means that those doctors who do not push their patients into being vaccinated are financially penalised.

It is not the purpose of this book to examine in depth the arguments against immunisation; there are several excellent books which do this, (see the Suggested Reading on page 78). There are also a growing number of organisations that can provide support if you believe your child has been damaged by vaccination, or if you are seeking more information about the vaccination debate (see page 78).

It is evident that there are a growing number of people who are convinced by the arguments against vaccination and who are choosing not to vaccinate themselves or their children. Or they may wish to give their child one or two immunisations, eg polio, but not the entire and ever-increasing number. There are also significant groups of people for whom vaccinations are contraindicated by the manufacturers themselves, eg pregnant women are not supposed to receive vaccinations against Hepatitis B or Yellow Fever as they may cause damage to the foetus.

CHAPTER 2

HOMŒOPATHY

The word 'homœopathy' comes from the Greek, and means 'similar suffering'. This points to the underlying principle of homœopathy which is that you can use the same thing to restore balance that created the imbalance, or use 'like to cure like'. Whilst this underlying principle has been known since ancient times, homœopathy in the form that we use it now has only been developed in the last two hundred years.

A German physician, Samuel Hahnemann, developed homœopathy in the late eighteenth century after discovering that he got better results when he gave more and more minute substances of a medicine than when he gave the usual large doses. A homœopathic remedy is not just a minute dose, however, it has also gone through a process of potentisation whereby the substance is repeatedly banged or 'succussed' to release its full healing potential.

The homœopathic remedy restores health by providing a stimulus to the natural healing mechanisms within us all. It is paradoxical to our materialistic way of thinking that the more times the substance is diluted, the higher the potency, and the more profound the effects of the remedy. Do not let this put you off trying homœopathy; it works on adults, children and animals, whether or not we believe in it.

Homœopathic remedies are chosen by matching the most appropriate remedy 'picture' to that of the sufferer. This is done by accurate and careful observation of the person. Note as many symptoms as you can and use them as clues to finding the right remedy.

There are no side effects to homœopathic remedies. If you do keep taking the remedy day after day for a long period of time you may begin to take on some of the symptoms of the remedy, in which case you should simply stop taking them. This situation should not arise, however, as remedies should only be taken when required for prophylaxis or treatment.

We call the method of taking homœopathic remedies to prevent a disease homœopathic prophylaxis. The idea is that you take a particular remedy into your system so that it is ready to act should you come into contact with the corresponding disease. The disease will therefore not get a chance to establish itself and you will not experience any symptoms. If the action of the remedy isn't needed the body simply doesn't utilise it.

Homœopathic prophylaxis has a very good success rate and many examples of its efficacy are to be found in homœopathic books. An eminent homœopath Dorothy Shepherd states that the homœopathic remedy *Pertussin* was given daily for two weeks to 364 cases after contact with whooping cough and not one child developed the disease. Leslie Speight writes of another physician who gave *Lathyrus sativa* to 82 people who were in close proximity to a polio outbreak with 12 people being direct contacts and not one developed the disease. There are many accounts in current farming journals of homœopathic vets getting excellent results by giving farm animals homœopathic nosodes to prevent common farm diseases. However, there is never any absolute guarantee that you will not get a disease, whatever measures you take, because there is always a possibility that you are exceptionally susceptible to a particular disease, or if your immune system is already under strain then you will be more susceptible to any disease.

Prophylactic remedies may be one of the range of homœopathic remedies made from plants, animal products or minerals, or they may be a special type of remedy known as a nosode. Nosodes are actually made from diseased body tissue or discharges such as sputum. In common with any other homœopathic remedy, the process of potentisation renders them chemically harmless but homœopathically active. Where a choice has been offered in the Disease Section of this book between a remedy and a nosode, both have been proven to be effective in preventing the disease, and you should take whichever is most readily available or what your homœopath advises.

If any disease symptoms do develop then try the most clearly indicated homœopathic remedy. Under the disease headings you will see a list of the homœopathic remedies most commonly used for treating that disease. Compare these remedies by looking them up in the Materia Medica section of this book, and take the one that seems to fit your symptoms the best. Generally it is best to try one remedy for a day and if there is no benefit then try the next best indicated one. If the deterioration of health is very rapid then do not wait for a whole day but change the remedy if there is no response after a few hours. It is not uncommon for one remedy to be appropriate for one stage of an illness and for a different remedy to be needed at a later stage.

If it is possible to establish a link with an experienced homœopath in your area before becoming ill, and particularly if you have young children, then it is advisable to do so. Choosing the right homœopathic remedy can be straightforward, but there are also times when it can be confusing and then professional advice may be necessary to get a good response, (to find a homœopath see the list of Contacts in the Appendix).

POTENCY

Homœopathic remedies are prepared by a system which involves dilution and potentisation. An amount of the original substance is taken, mixed with alcohol and made into a tincture (Mother Tincture).

The letter C which may follow the remedy that you purchase stands for centesimal scale. This means that one hundredth of the Mother Tincture is taken out and added to another ninety-nine parts of alcohol, it is shaken (succussed) and this results in a 1C remedy. This is done 30 times to produce a 30C remedy. By custom the letter C (centesimal) is often omitted, so the remedy *Sulphur* 30, is in fact *Sulphur* in the 30th centesimal potency.

A 6X remedy is based on a different method of division, known as the decimal scale. One part in ten is taken out each time and added to another ten parts. In parts of Europe, the suffix X is replaced by the prefix D. Thus,

Sulphur 6X is the same as *Sulphur* D6.

As stated above, the more diluted the remedy, then the more potent is its action. This means that *Sulphur* 30C has a more profound action than *Sulphur* 6C; also that *Sulphur* 6C has a more profound action than *Sulphur* 6X. Remedies that are made from poisons are not usually available in potencies under 6C because there is a chance that a tiny amount of the original substance may be left in the very low potency remedies.

DOSAGE:

Prophylactic remedies are most commonly taken in the 30th potency (30C or 30 centesimal). The potency and dosage is advised under the prophylaxis heading of each disease section.

The 6th and 30th centesimal potency are the most commonly available homœopathic remedies and they are suitable for treating most acute illnesses. Generally speaking, the more severe the symptoms then the higher the potency that you take.

A lower potency should be given more often than a higher, eg. give a 6th potency every two to four hours but a 30th potency every eight to twelve hours. If using the 200th potency then only one dose should be taken and only repeated after a time if absolutely necessary. Potencies higher than 200 should only be taken on professional advice.

Once the condition improves then STOP taking the remedy. If the symptoms return then repeat the remedy. If the symptom picture changes then change the remedy.

TAKING THE REMEDY

Homœopathic remedies are available as tablets, granules, powders and liquids. Tablets are the most easily managed, but granules are less bulky for travellers. One tablet or a couple of granules constitutes one dose. This is more than adequate to initiate a healing response and you will not get a stronger effect by taking a larger amount. An increase in the medicinal action of a remedy can only be obtained by either taking it more frequently or by taking a higher potency.

The remedy should be placed under your tongue and allowed to dissolve. Do not eat, drink, smoke or use toothpaste for twenty minutes before or after taking a remedy. Try not to handle the remedy, but shake one dose into the lid of the bottle and then drop that straight into your mouth. For infants a tablet may be crushed between two clean teaspoons and then tipped into the mouth.

It is advisable to avoid taking coffee and strong smelling substances such as camphor and eucalyptus whilst using a homœopathic treatment as they may antidote it. No harm will be produced by combining homœopathic with orthodox drugs although it may mean that the homœopathic remedy does not work so effectively.

Store your remedies in their original container away from strong smells and out of the light. Do not expose homœopathic remedies to X-Rays as this may reduce their effectiveness; ask airport officials to look at them rather than having them X-Rayed with your luggage. Homœopathic remedies are legally transportable across international borders.

CHAPTER 3

PLANT MEDICINE

Herbal medicine is part of our traditional and ancient wisdom. We are very fortunate that this wisdom has not been totally lost following the introduction of synthetic drug treatments.

Many of our modern drugs have been synthesised by basing the chemistry on a particular component of a plant medicine. It is now being realised, however, that individual constituents of a plant do not have the same effect as the whole plant for a number of reasons. Firstly, every plant has an enormous number of constituents, only some of which will have been analysed and several of these will probably be working together synergistically to achieve an effect. This is why many herbs are actually more effective in the long run than drug treatments which tend to give dramatic but only short-lived benefit. Secondly, components isolated from a plant or synthesised tend to be extremely powerful and damaging whereas in their natural state their effect is often 'buffered' by other constituents within the plant. These factors support the idea that plants are not beneficial for us by chance, but because they, as we, are part of an intricate web of interdependence.

How can plants prevent infectious disease? Protection may be achieved in two ways; firstly by utilising the antiseptic properties of plants, and secondly by using them to support the bodily systems. The highly antiseptic properties of plants are most usually found in the volatile components and thus essential oils are extremely useful here. Supporting the bodily system will often require taking the herb internally, as an infusion, tincture, capsule, etc.

ESSENTIAL OILS

Essential oils are essences extracted from the flowers, leaves, barks, roots and fruit of plants. When you squeeze a piece of orange peel, the fragrant droplets you can see are an essential oil that was contained in little sacs within the peel. The most common way to extract essential oils is by steam distillation, although other methods are used for certain other plants.

Essential oils have been used for thousands of years as natural antiseptics. In more recent years this bactericidal action has been attributed to the fact that essential oils are naturally rich in phenols, alcohols, esters, acids and aldehydes. Several of these constituents have been isolated for use as medical antiseptics; however, as is so often the case, the whole has proved to be greater than the sum of the parts, and the essential oil itself is more effective against a wide spectrum of disease agents than the isolated components or synthetic derivatives such as phenol. The other advantages of essential oils are that they are effective in minute concentrations and their effect lasts for a longer time.

The essential oils that have the most effective anti-microbial properties for general use are: *Cinnamon, Clove, Eucalyptus, Lavender, Lemon, Pine, Tea Tree* and *Thyme.*

For personal use, a number of the oils may be applied to the skin. This will be useful when you are in the company of another person suspected to have an infectious disease, or when travelling through an epidemic area. Essential oils, with one or two exceptions, should not be applied to the skin undiluted. Many of the oils are skin irritants when concentrated and several of them should never be applied to the skin even when diluted.

Antiseptic oils which may be diluted and applied to the skin include: *Eucalyptus, Lavender, Lemon, Pine, Tea Tree* and *Thyme.* These may be diluted in a carrier or base oil, such as almond, soya or grapeseed oil. The oils may be used in combination but the combination of essential oils should not exceed a strength of more than 2% in a base oil. This means that to a 100ml of base oil, you can add up to 2ml or approximately 60 drops of essential oils. The prepared oil may be massaged onto the skin; alternatively you can add 5 to 10 drops of any of these oils to a bath. If you have sensitive skin you should always do a patch test before applying a new substance.

The essential oils of *Lavender* and *Tea Tree* are very unlikely to be an irritant and most people find that they can apply these to the skin undiluted without any adverse reaction. *Lavender* is particularly useful for healing and soothing burns and should be poured on to the burn as soon as possible to prevent blistering and infection. *Tea Tree* is a highly antiseptic and antiviral essential oil that may be poured onto any wound to prevent infection, it also has the advantage of not stinging, unlike many other antiseptic preparations. These two essential oils make up an invaluable part of any first-aid kit.

If you do get an infectious disease then essential oils may also be used therapeutically to help you fight off the illness and recover more quickly. In this situation, you can either spray the room you are in or use a burner, apply the prepared massage oil or have steam inhalations. Applying massage oil to the abdomen will be useful for diseases of the intestinal tract such as those that cause diarrhoea. Steam inhalations will be very beneficial for diseases of the respiratory tract such as measles, influenza or whooping cough.

To prepare a steam inhalation take a bowl of hot water and add a few drops of essential oil. The oils of *Eucalyptus, Lemon, Pine, Tea Tree* and *Thyme* are particularly good as inhalations. Combinations of two or more oils may also be used. Place a towel to cover your head and then lean over the bowl so that you can inhale the vapours for a few minutes. Do not use *Eucalyptus* if you are also taking homœopathic remedies as it may antidote the homœopathic treatment.

Essential oils may also be used to fumigate a sick-room. Fill a plant spray with water and add twenty drops of each of the oils that you have available, (You do not need to use all the oils, three or four in combination will be adequate) then spray the room thoroughly every few hours. Essential oils suitable to use in a room spray include *Cinnamon, Clove,*

Eucalyptus, Lavender, Lemon and *Pine.* Not only will the airborne spray kill off disease pathogens in the room, but this method has also been shown to have a therapeutic effect on the patient. This is because as well as having a marked antimicrobial effect, several of the oils stimulate the cells and organs involved in the immune response. Essential oils that best combine the antiseptic and immune stimulant actions include: *Eucalyptus, Lavender, Lemon* and *Tea Tree.*

Alternatively you can buy an essential oil burner which will use a candle flame or a light bulb to heat a plate. A few drops of essential oil are added to the hot plate and the vapours will fumigate the room

Essential oils have also long been used as insect repellents. They seem to work by masking body smells into something less attractive to insects. The chief remedy for repelling mosquitoes is *Citronella* although *Eucalyptus, Lemon* and *Lemon Grass* may also be of help.These may be diluted in a base oil or *Witchazel* lotion and applied to the skin. Alternatively, a traditional method in parts of North Africa is to burn *Citronella* on an essential oil burner in the room.

MEDICINAL HERBS

The use of plants as medicine has evolved with mankind from ancient times and is a knowledge that has been handed down in every culture. Using herbs to prevent and treat infectious illness can be very effective although success will often depend on a detailed knowledge of the appropriate herbs to use. There are, however, certain herbs that have the ability to generally strengthen the immune response and these may be safely used for our purpose of preventing and alleviating infectious diseases.

The herbs that are of most interest to us here are those that fit into the categories known as adaptogens and alteratives. Adaptogens are substances that help us to deal with or adapt to stresses in our environment. They work by helping to improve or maintain hormonal secretions, particularly those of the adrenal cortex, that enable us to cope with physical and psychological stress. In the past such herbs were known as tonics. One of the best known adaptogens is *Ginseng,* which is a useful remedy for anybody who is feeling run down and vulnerable to becoming ill. *Ginseng* is not appropriate to take actually during an acute illness as it is too warming, but it is useful to take to help prevent illness, particularly in the elderly, when feeling depleted of energy or during convalescence.

Many adaptogens may seem to have contradictory actions as they have a normalising or balancing effect on a bodily system, rather than forcing the system to react in a particular way. Useful examples are *Dandelion* and *Wormwood* for the digestive system, *Chelidonium* for the liver, *Garlic* for the small intestine, *Boneset* and *Yarrow* for the fever mechanism, and *Mullein* and *White Horehound* for the respiratory tract. This means that these herbs will be beneficial to take for any ailment involving one of these particular bodily systems, and they may also be taken to strengthen that bodily system if you know that you have a weakness in that area.

Alteratives promote health by helping to detoxify and purify the bodily systems, they may also have an anti-microbial action. Alteratives used to be known as 'blood cleansers'. The most useful alterative herbs for the prevention or treatment of infectious diseases are *Echinacea* and *Garlic*. *Garlic* is best taken by eating the raw clove on a regular basis.

Echinacea is such a useful herb that it is worth a special mention. *Echinacea* is the principal anti-microbial herb. It is both a natural antibiotic and is very effective at strengthening the immune system. For this reason *Echinacea* is invaluable in the treatment and prevention of all infectious diseases. It is active against both viral and bacterial disease pathogens. *Echinacea* tincture or capsules can be taken daily for up to three months when travelling in high risk areas, or take for three weeks as soon any symptoms of an infectious disease develop.

Where herbs are known to have a beneficial effect in the treatment of a particular disease, they have been recommended under the treatment section of that disease. The herbs that have been recommended here are available throughout Europe and North America. These herbs will be effective wherever you are, but obviously you must be able to take sufficient a supply with you. Every part of the world has developed its own system of herbal medicine based on local plants and appropriate to local conditions. In fact, herbal medicine is the most widely taken form of medicine in the world. If you are spending sufficient time in another country to get acquainted with the local herbal practices then this will be the most practical and valuable thing to do.

DOSAGE

Herbal remedies are usually taken three times a day. In a very acute situation, eg. influenza, you may wish to take the remedy more frequently.

When treating an acute illness, just take the herbs for a few days until the symptoms pass. For symptoms that drag on following an illness, most herbs may be taken safely for up to six weeks. If any symptoms remain after that time you should consult a practitioner.

Directions on how to take the herbs follow. For children halve the dosages, for children under four years quarter the dosages. Do not take any herbs in therapeutic doses during pregnancy without first checking with a practitioner.

HOW TO TAKE HERBAL REMEDIES

Infusions: An infusion is made like a tea. Use this method for the softer, green or flowering parts of the plant. Place the herb in a pot, pour on boiling water and leave to steep for ten minutes before straining. A general guide to quantity is to use one or two teaspoonfuls of the dried herb or herb mixture to a cupful of boiling water. Quantities will vary according to the freshness and quality of the herb used and the strength of the infusion required.

Decoctions: Use this method for the harder or woodier roots, barks, berries or seeds of a plant. Using a similar quantity as for an infusion, place the plant material in a saucepan, pour on the water, cover the pot and then bring to the boil and simmer for ten to fifteen minutes before straining. If steam escapes add a little more water.

Tinctures: The most convenient way of taking a herb, a tincture is an extraction of the herb using water and alcohol. A standard dose is 5ml of tincture in a wineglass of water three times a day.

PART II

THE
DISEASES

CHOLERA

Cholera is a disease of the gastro-intestinal tract that tends to occur in epidemics. It is spread by faecally contaminated food and water, and by flies. In the developed world cholera has disappeared due to the improved sanitation and hygiene.

The incubation period is two to five days. The symptoms include nausea, vomiting, abdominal cramps and severe watery diarrhoea ('rice-water' stools). The diarrhoea causes dehydration and a fall in blood pressure and fatalities are most often from circulatory failure.

The cholera vaccine is notoriously ineffective, at best offering 50% protection and then only for a few months. Under orthodox treatment the mortality rate is still about 50%. Cholera is a disease where homœopathy has been spectacularly successful with mortality rates in Europe during the outbreaks of the 1850s at 5-9%.

HOMŒOPATHIC PROPHYLAXIS
Cholera 30 (nosode): one prior to travelling and once a week during an outbreak.

or

Cuprum 30: once a week during an outbreak.

TREATMENT
Homœopathic: *Camphor, Cuprum, Veratrum alb*

DIPHTHERIA

Diphtheria is an infectious disease with a short incubation period (two to four days). Due to improved hygiene it is now rare in developed countries, but is still significant in the developing world. Children are mostly affected, although during epidemics it may also be seen in adults. Many adults are naturally immune and immunity can be established by a skin test. Immunisation against diphtheria is part of the DPT vaccine given routinely to infants.

Symptoms start with a sore throat and the tonsils and larynx or sometimes the nose may become affected. The tonsils become covered with a greyish-white membrane that may extend over the soft palate and cannot be wiped off with a swab. It has a musty, sickening smell. In severe cases the membrane may obstruct the larynx and breathing becomes obstructed. A generalised toxaemia may also develop causing a fall in blood pressure or paralysis. Any suspicion of paralysis should be referred to a doctor urgently as this can also affect the ability to breathe.

Reports as to the efficacy of the immunisation vary greatly. Serious side effects including death from anaphylactic shock are well documented.

HOMŒOPATHIC PROPHYLAXIS

Diphtherinum 30 (nosode): Once a week during risk of infection.

or

Pyrogen 30: Once a week during risk of infection.

TREATMENT

Homœopathic: *Apis, Arsenicum, Lac caninum, Lachesis, Mercurius, Phytolacca, Pyrogen.*

HEPATITIS

Infectious hepatitis is an acute inflammation of the liver associated with a virus infection. Two strains of virus have been identified known as Hepatitis A and Hepatitis B.

Hepatitis A is usually transmitted via food or drink contaminated with infected faecal matter and is most common in areas where sanitation is poor. The incubation period is 3 to 6 weeks. Hepatitis A is nearly always a self-limiting disease with a complete recovery usual and a low mortality rate (less than 0.2%). Very occasionally the case is fulminating, with delirium, high fever and intense jaundice and without correct treatment these cases may be fatal.

Hepatitis B (HB) is also known as serum hepatitis, and is contacted via inadequately sterilised syringes and needles, poor surgical technique and sexual contact. The incubation period is 3 to 6 months.

High risk groups for contracting Hepatitis B are intravenous drug users, the sexually promiscuous, and health care workers who handle bodily fluids.

Some countries have instated a routine Hepatitis B vaccination schedule for all children regardless of whether or not they are at a high risk of contracting the disease. In 1998 the French Health Minister announced that they were suspending hepatitis B vaccinations for schoolchildren, four years after a mass immunisation began, 'because of fears the vaccine could cause neurological disorders, in particular multiple sclerosis'. (Associated Press report, October 1998). Immunisation is also offered to travellers.

The symptoms of hepatitis develop over a few days and are marked by a loss of appetite and nausea especially on the sight of food, and particularly fatty food. There is a general feeling of malaise and there may be a headache. After a few days of these symptoms the urine becomes dark and the faeces pale. The conjunctiva of the eyes and the skin become yellow as jaundice develops.

Even mild cases of hepatitis should rest in bed as this lessens the damage to the liver and hastens recovery. The diet must be very light with no fats and no alcohol. Alcohol, drugs and rich foods should be avoided for many months following hepatitis to allow the liver to recover. Professional treatment is advised, particularly in severe cases.

Immunisation is not advised for pregnant women.

HOMŒOPATHIC PROPHYLAXIS
Hepatitis A 30: Once a week in high risk areas.
Hepatitis B 30: Three doses 12 hours apart following a high risk incident such as a dubious injection or operation.

HERBAL PROPHYLAXIS
Chelidonium: Particularly useful when travelling in high risk areas or if you know your liver function is poor. Take 5 drops of the tincture in a little water three times a day during travel. If Chelidonium tincture is unavailable take the homœopathic remedy in low potency eg. 6X, once a day.

TREATMENT
Homœopathic: *Lycopodium, Natrum Sulph, Phosphorus*
Herbal: *Boldo, Dandelion Root, Milk Thistle*
These herbs will assist the liver to heal. Combine the herbs and make an infusion to drink three times a day for up to six weeks.

INFLUENZA ('FLU)

Influenza is an infection of the respiratory tract often accompanied with symptoms of aching and feverishness. Different strains of influenza will cause different symptoms including sore throats, coughs and gastric disorders.

Influenza normally lasts from two to five days but more serious complications can develop, particularly in the elderly. There seems to be an increasing tendency for influenza symptoms to linger, leaving the person feeling debilitated and depressed afterwards.

Immunisation is carried out, particularly on the elderly, at the beginning of the winter. Because there are so many different strains of influenza their effectiveness is very limited, and there is also evidence that they reduce the general immunity making the person more vulnerable to other illnesses.

HOMŒOPATHIC PROPHYLAXIS
Influenzinum 30 (nosode): One dose three times a week during an epidemic. It is possible to get a specific influenza strain as a remedy if you have time to request your pharmacist following an outbreak eg. Influenzinum Beijing.
　　or
Aconite, Gelsemium & Eupatorium 30 (combination remedy): An excellent combination remedy to take as a prophylactic or as soon as any 'flu symptoms develop. One dose every twelve hours for three days following contact with the disease or eight hourly starting immediately any 'flu symptoms develop.

TREATMENT
Homœopathic: *Aconite, Ars alb, Bryonia, Eupatorium, Gelsemium, Rhus tox*
Herbal: *Boneset, Elderflower, Peppermint, Yarrow*
A combination of herbs that are decongestant and help to balance the fever mechanism. Combine and make an infusion to drink every four hours until the fever symptoms pass. Omit the *Peppermint* if you are also taking homœopathic remedies as it may antidote the treatment.
Take *Echinacea* for up to six weeks if any symptoms linger.

MALARIA

Four species of the malarial parasite infect man, and they are all carried by mosquitoes of the genus Anopheles, which flourish in tropical and subtropical countries.

The risk of contracting malaria varies according to the season and locality, for more information contact the Malaria Reference Library Helpline (0891-600350) before travelling. The most effective way to avoid malaria is to prevent yourself from being bitten by mosquitoes; wear protective clothing, use insect repellents and sleep under a mosquito net.

The main symptoms of malaria are a headache, fever and rigor (shivering fit). Jaundice and general malaise may develop. A blood test should be taken to confirm diagnosis. Most common is 'benign' malaria which is characterised by intermittent fevers which may recur from time to time for several years. The mortality rate of benign malaria in previously healthy people is low. 'Malignant' malaria, which is more common in West Africa, although it is also found elsewhere, is characterised by profound jaundice and profound anæmia and urgent professional treatment must be sought as the mortality rate of this type of malaria is high.

Orally administered drugs are the orthodox technique for attempting to avoid malaria. The malarial parasites are increasingly resistant to these drugs and they should not be taken during pregnancy. Anti-malarial drugs can also cause a number of well-reported side effects including drowsiness, headaches, visual disturbances and tinnitus.

HOMŒOPATHIC PROPHYLAXIS

No remedies, orthodox or alternative, can guarantee prevention of Malaria. However, the risk and severity of an attack can be lessened with appropriate prophylaxis.

Malaria 30 (nosode): once a week in high risk areas. Continue for four weeks after leaving a high risk area.
 and
China officinalis 6: take once a day for the other 6 days of the week in high risk areas. Continue for two weeks after leaving a high risk area.

TREATMENT

Homœopathic Remedies: *Arsenicum alb, China off, Eupatorium, Natrum mur, Pulsatilla, Sulphur*

MEASLES

Measles is one of the classic childhood illnesses. The early symptoms are a sore throat, cold symptoms, inflamed eyes, a cough and feverishness. On about the fourth day a rash appears on the child's neck and behind the ears, which gradually moves downwards to cover the body. Most children recover fully without treatment after about ten days. The incubation period is ten to twelve days and the most infectious period just before the rash appears.

Very occasionally complications develop usually caused by dehydration from a high fever, or difficulty breathing due to a secondary chest infection. Contrary to the popular myth there is no danger of permanent eye damage except in situations where vitamin A is deficient. Very rarely a more serious complication involving inflammation of the brain tissues (encephalitis) may develop. Seek urgent medical treatment if there are any signs of unusual drowsiness, a severe headache or marked irritability. Encephalitis is most likely to result from 'atypical' measles which is more common in children immunised against measles.

In 1994 a study showed a possible connection between the measles inoculation and the sharp rise in Crohn's disease and colitis in children. (The Lancet, 1994, 343: 105). The measles vaccine has also been known to cause deaths from infection, thrombocytopenia, fatal shock, and in a Danish study to cause arthritis and dermatitis.

According to traditional Chinese medicine, measles, along with the other classic childhood diseases, offers the child an opportunity to throw off any toxins that may have accumulated during pregnancy. Immunisation denies the child the opportunity to clear out these poisons. A study on African children has shown that those who catch measles tend to suffer less from allergic conditions, such as asthma, eczema and hay fever.

General home care includes bed rest, sponging down with tepid water during the fever stage and soothing the itchy rash with the gentle herbal remedies listed overleaf.

HOMŒOPATHIC PROPHYLAXIS

Morbillinum 30 (nosode): It may be better to allow your child to contract measles and get it over with. If your child is very weak and it is inadvisable to contract measles then take one dose of this remedy if he/she comes into contact with the disease. This remedy may also be given to clear up a severe or lingering case of measles.

TREATMENT

Homœopathic Remedies: *Belladonna, Euphrasia, Pulsatilla* (most common), *Rhus tox*

HERBAL REMEDIES:

Internal: *Boneset, Chamomile, Eyebright*

Combine the herbs to make a soothing and decongestant infusion to drink three times a day until the symptoms pass.

External: *Chamomile, Chickweed*

Make an infusion of these two soothing herbs and when cool use to sponge over the rash

MENINGITIS

Meningitis means inflammation of the meninges, which are the membranes surrounding the brain and the spinal cord. The most common organism causing infectious meningitis is the meningococcus.

Most people who become infected with the meningococcus organism confine it to their throat and recover without developing other symptoms. In certain situations the organism may enter the bloodstream and then the symptoms of meningitis rapidly develop.

Meningitis used to be a disease prevalent in certain parts of the Third World and amongst those subject to a damp and overcrowded environment. Other than this it was very rare. In the past few years there has been a growth in the number of outbreaks of meningitis in the UK, particularly in children. Reasons for this increase are only speculative but it may be another indication that the immune system of children subjected to an increasing number of stresses such as environmental pollutants and inoculations is no longer able to fight off infectious diseases.

The symptoms of meningitis are due to the inflammation of the meninges causing increased intracranial pressure. The onset is sudden with the patient becoming severely ill and with a high fever. There is a severe and persistent headache which may be associated with vomiting. The person is drowsy and irritable. They tend to lie in a characteristic attitude which is curled up and turned away from the light, as photophobia is present. They resent being touched or disturbed and, if a child, cry with a high-pitched cry. There is a marked stiffness of the neck, and any attempt to flex the head is strongly resisted. Convulsions or fits are common in infants. In meningococcal meningitis there is often a skin rash.

If treated rapidly, before a coma develops, then the recovery rate of infectious meningitis is high. But speed is essential and immediate medical treatment must be sought as any delay makes complications more likely.

Inoculation used to be confined to those coming into direct contact with a person having meningitis. In 1987, in New Zealand, the Health Department began a trial of vaccinating children against meningitis. However, the high incidence of adverse effects led to a public outcry and the abandonment of the trial.

In the UK, since 1992, there has been a move to inoculate all infants routinely against meningitis with the Haemophilus influenzae type b (or Hib) vaccine. This type of bacterial meningitis effects mainly pre-school children, and the risk appears to be higher in child-care facilities which cater for very young infants that are not toilet trained. There are thought to be approximately 20 deaths a year in the UK from Hib. Reports on the effectiveness of the Hib vaccine vary, in the UK it is regarded as 65-74% effective, (The Lancet, 1991, 338: 395-8).

The meningitis inoculation should not be carried out on pregnant women or those already suffering from an inflammatory illness such as influenza.

HOMŒOPATHIC PROPHYLAXIS

Meningococcus 30 (nosode): Take this following any contact with the disease. One dose in the morning three times a week for two weeks. Other nosodes are available if it is known that a different organism is responsible for the outbreak.

and

Belladonna 30: One dose in the evening three times a week for two weeks.

TREATMENT

If any symptoms indicating the possibility of meningitis develop get immediate professional treatment. While waiting for a prescription or test results take *Belladonna* 30 every four hours.

MUMPS

Mumps is caused by a virus infection and is one of the common childhood diseases. The characteristic symptom is a swelling of one or both of the salivary glands (parotids) just below and in front of the ears. Other symptoms include feverishness and a sore throat. No particular treatment is necessary as mumps in children is not a serious illness. The swelling usually begins to go down after two or three days.

In recent years the immunisation against mumps is performed on infants as part of the MMR vaccine. This is promoted on the basis that although mumps is not a serious illness for children, it may cause orchitis, a swelling of the testicles, in adult men. There is a commonly held belief that mumps contracted by an adult male will result in sterility; this is actually extremely rare as nearly all cases clear up totally and usually only one testicle is affected.

It makes far more sense for boys to get mumps before they become adults as then sterility cannot occur. In fact, it is not known whether or not protection from the mumps vaccine lasts into adulthood, whereas having mumps as a child nearly always provides protection as an adult.

The reported side effects of the MMR vaccine include allergic reactions, febrile seizures, nerve deafness and more rarely, encephelitis.

HOMŒOPATHIC PROPHYLAXIS

Parotidinum 30 (nosode): It is advisable to allow children to contract mumps however this remedy may be given to adult males who did not have mumps as a child. One dose after coming into contact with the disease and one dose the following week.

TREATMENT

Homœopathic: *Apis, Belladonna, Mercurius, Phytolacca, Pulsatilla*

Herbal: *Balm, Chamomile, Yarrow*

Combine the herbs and make a soothing infusion to drink three times a day until the symptoms pass.

POLIO

Poliomyelitis is caused by a virus infection which specifically attacks nerve cells in the spinal cord. The virus grows in the intestinal tract and is excreted in the faeces, the incubation period is 7 to 14 days. Whereas polio is still a significant disease in areas where sanitation is neglected and hygiene is poor, in western countries polio is now an extremely rare disease. The oral polio vaccine is given routinely to infants.

The early symptoms of poliomyelitis include a headache, sore throat and stiffness of the neck and back. In most cases the disease progresses no further and unless there is a polio epidemic it is often mistaken for influenza. If the full-blown disease sets in then on the fourth or fifth day paralysis develops and proceeds to its full extent in about 36 hours. The paralysis usually affects the limbs and the muscles become painful and tender, beginning to waste about 3 weeks after the onset of paralysis. If the muscles of respiration are affected breathing may become hampered. Rarely polio may also affect the brain causing encephelitis.

It is important that anyone suspected of having polio rests in bed as paralysis is more likely to occur in muscles which are kept active. If necessary artificial aids to breathing are used. After about three weeks the muscles may be gradually moved and most will begin to recover at this time. Most people make a full recovery from polio although fatalities do occur due to pneumonia or circulatory collapse. Physiotherapy should be continued for up to 6 months as muscle recovery can continue through this period.

The effectiveness of the polio immunisation in reducing the incidence of polio is controversial. There have been three polio epidemics in the USA this century. The first two declined when there was no treatment offered, in the late 1940s the decline of the third epidemic was credited to the polio vaccine although this has since been disputed.

In recent years the inoculation against polio is the most common cause of polio in the developed world, as even the so called 'dead' vaccine (Salk type) can cause polio. Also polio is excreted in the stools of those just vaccinated for approximately six weeks afterwards, and there have been a small number of cases of parents contracting polio after changing the nappies of recently immunised infants. Thus special attention should be paid to hygiene during nappy changes. There is no evidence that public swimming pools spread polio in this way, most likely because the chlorine or other disinfectants in the water kill the virus.

The polio vaccine has been held responsible for cases of encephalitis and Guillain-Barre syndrome, which causes paralysis. Polio vaccines also contain small amounts of a number of antibiotics and those with a hypersensitivity to antibiotics should avoid the vaccine. The vaccine should not be given during pregnancy.

HOMŒOPATHIC PROPHYLAXIS
Poliomyelitis 30 (nosode): One dose a week for three weeks if there is an epidemic or contact with the disease is suspected.
　or
Lathyrus 30: One dose a week for three weeks following any contact with the disease.

TREATMENT
Homœopathic: *Gelsemium, Lathyrus*

RUBELLA (GERMAN MEASLES)

German measles is a harmless disease in children causing symptoms of slight feverishness, nasal discharge and a rash of small, slightly raised spots that tend to move down the body. The duration is about three days or less.

Rubella is a potential threat to pregnant women, since those who contract it during the first three months of pregnancy are considered to have approximately a 10% risk of having a baby with birth defects, including blindness, deafness, a heart condition, cleft palate or mental problems. It is for this reason that inoculation is given to infants as part of the MMR injection. However the immunity offered by inoculation does not last into adulthood whereas contracting German measles as a child usually does, so it would offer more protection to expose your daughter to German measles as a child.

There is a blood test that can check for natural immunity to rubella which can be easily carried out by your GP for any woman concerned. Side effects to the MMR vaccine are well recorded including convulsions, allergic reactions and rarely encephalitis.

HOMŒOPATHIC PROPHYLAXIS

Rubella 30: May be taken by any pregnant woman who comes into contact with the disease. One dose three times a week for three weeks.

TREATMENT

Homœopathic: *Belladonna, Mercurius, Pulsatilla*
Herbal: *Boneset, Chamomile, Elderflower*
Combine the herbs and make an infusion to drink three times a day to relieve any symptoms of feverishness or discomfort.

TETANUS

Tetanus is caused by bacteria which usually enter the body through wounds, especially deep penetrating wounds, eg. from a nail. The bacillus is most commonly present in soil and especially horse manure and so cleaning wounds thoroughly, particularly if infected with soil, is of the utmost importance in preventing the disease.

The main symptoms are severe muscular spasms that usually start in the jaw muscles, causing difficulty in opening the mouth – lockjaw. The spasms then spread to other muscles so that severe spasms become generalised. Orthodox treatment is to combine sedation and curare with large doses of tetanus anti-toxin.

The tetanus immunisation has caused death due to anaphylactic shock and also cases of Guillain-Barre syndrome, which causes paralysis. It is given routinely to infants as part of the DPT vaccine, and also advised by the orthodox health system regularly for adults.

HOMŒOPATHIC PROPHYLAXIS

Clostridium tetani 30 (nosode): Take once a week during high risk activities, ie. trekking, mountaineering, exploring. Or one dose twice a week for three weeks following a deep, penetrating wound.

or

Ledum 30: One dose three times in one week following any suspect wound or animal bite.

TUBERCULOSIS

Tuberculosis (TB) is caused by the tubercle bacillus, Mycobacterium tuberculosis. The two types which can effect man are the human or the bovine type. The human type usually infects the lungs; the bovine type usually infects children and causes inflammation of the lymph glands and the bones. The bovine type was spread by ingesting milk, and has virtually disappeared due to improved public hygiene, the pasteurisation of milk and the prevention of tuberculosis in cattle.

The human type, also called pulmonary tuberculosis, is spread by infected sputum and by coughing. The most important single factor in the spread of pulmonary tuberculosis worldwide is overcrowding; there is a direct correlation between the increase in standards of living and a fall in the incidence of tuberculosis. Tuberculosis had virtually died out in the developed world, however the past few years has seen a small increase in the number of cases, particularly in overcrowded neighbourhoods of British inner cities.

Despite a very active worldwide vaccination campaign, pulmonary tuberculosis is still prevalent in tropical countries, and the incidence is higher in recent immigrants from those parts of the world, and in people who travel there. There also seems to be a link between TB and AIDS, since the same groups with a high incidence of HIV and AIDS also have a high incidence of TB.

In Britain, the BCG vaccine is given at birth to Asian and other immigrant families; to those who live in or travel to areas of high risk; those in contact with active TB; and those with a family history of TB in the past five years. As well as these high risk groups, it is also offered to all British school-children between the ages of 10 and 14.

The effectiveness of the BCG vaccine varies greatly around the world, from zero to 80%. This variation is possibly due to strain variations, genetic or nutritional differences, and to environmental influences (The Lancet, 1995, 346: 1339-45). Side effects of the vaccine may include disseminated TB in immunosuppressed individuals, local ulceration, osteitis, lymphadenitis and generalised lymphadenopathy. (Medical Monitor, June 5, 1992).

Many children or young adults are infected with tubercle bacilli without any symptoms or obvious illness, and healing occurs naturally. The tuberculin test carried out prior to BCG vaccination in schools shows about one in ten to be tuberculin positive, in which case the vaccination is usually not given.

The symptoms of active pulmonary TB include generalised disorders such as weight loss, loss of appetite, malaise, low grade fever, night sweats and fatigue. There may also be a persistent cough, breathlessness, blood-stained sputum or the sudden coughing up of bright red blood.

Orthodox treatment of TB is with a combination of anti-tuberculous drugs. In the past few years a number of TB strains have emerged that are resistant to antibiotics.

HOMOEOPATHIC PROPHYLAXIS
Bacillinum 30 (nosode): Take one dose a week for three weeks following suspected exposure to the disease. If you experience prolonged exposure, ie through work, living conditions or travel then professional advice should be sought.

HOMOEOPATHIC TREATMENT
Treatment of tuberculosis will need ongoing supervision and probably a number of different remedies and should only be undertaken by a qualified practitioner. It should also be noted that it is illegal to treat tuberculosis other than by a Medical Doctor.

TYPHOID

Typhoid (enteric fever) is a disease of poor hygiene, being transmitted via the ingestion of contaminated food or water. It is most common in the tropics and subtropics. The disease organism affects the small intestine and whilst the symptoms are variable they generally begin with a fever and later severe diarrhoea develops.

There are a number of possible complications of typhoid including perforation of the intestine, pneumonia, meningitis and inflammation of the gall-bladder and hospital treatment is advisable.

The efficacy of the immunisation is not 100% and immunity wears off between 1 and 3 years. Severe side effects to the inoculation are not uncommon and it should not be performed on pregnant women, infants or when suffering from an inflammatory illness, eg influenza. Regular immunisations against typhoid can cause a hypersensitivity to the vaccine and these people must also avoid further immunisation.

HOMŒOPATHIC PROPHYLAXIS

Salmonella typhi 30 (nosode): Once a week when travelling in high risk areas.

TREATMENT

Homœopathic: *Arsenicum, Baptisia, Belladonna, Bryonia, Ipecac, Lachesis, Mercurius, Sulphur, Veratrum alb*

WHOOPING COUGH (PERTUSSIS)

Whooping cough is an infectious disease, usually occurring in children, which begins with symptoms of a common cold but after about a week a violent, convulsive cough, often followed by vomiting, occurs. The cough mainly occurs at night, but as the illness progresses it may appear during the day as well.

During a bout of coughing you may hear the characteristic 'whoop' as the child struggles to inhale. The child may cough as much as a dozen times with each breath, and their face may become blue. Whooping cough can be an exhausting and distressing experience for the parent and the child. Professional advice should be sought to treat whooping cough, especially in babies, and steps taken to avoid developing pneumonia or any damage to the lungs.

The vaccine against whooping cough is one of the most controversial of all immunisations. Cases of damaging side-effects are well documented, including skin conditions and convulsions leading to permanent brain damage or, in more rare cases, death. There are also serious doubts about the effectiveness of the inoculation and when immunisation was abandoned in Sweden and Germany due to concern about the potential side-effects, absolutely no increase in whooping cough cases occurred. In the UK the immunisation is still given routinely to infants as part of the DPT vaccine.

HOMŒOPATHIC PROPHYLAXIS
Pertussin 30 (nosode): Once a week during an epidemic or three doses in one week if your child has contact with the disease.

TREATMENT
Homœopathic: *Belladonna, Bryonia, Coccus cacti, Drosera, Ipecac*
Herbal: Aniseed, Coltsfoot, White Horehound, Thyme
Combine the herbs and make an infusion to drink three times a day until the symptoms pass. The infusion may also be sipped between bouts of coughing to reduce the severity.

YELLOW FEVER

Yellow fever is a viral disease endemic to tropical and subtropical Africa and America and with epidemics occurring elsewhere on occasion. It is transmitted by the bites of certain mosquitoes.

The incubation period is 3-6 days. Many mild cases of yellow fever occur with only a small percentage developing a severe form of the disease. Symptoms include fever, chills, aching muscles, headache, vomiting and pain in the upper abdomen with most cases clearing up at this stage. In severe cases the onset is more violent and jaundice and haemorrhages develop by about the fourth day. Severe cases can be fatal with mortality rates variable from 7-50%.

The inoculation is considered to be over 90% effective, however, it does affect the immune system detrimentally and is contraindicated for people taking steroids, and those with a history of allergies, cancer or who are HIV positive. The immunisation is also usually advised against for pregnant women and infants. An international certificate of vaccination against yellow fever is required when entering some countries. Taking precautions to avoid being bitten by mosquitoes which may carry the disease is essential in preventing the disease.

HOMŒOPATHIC PROPHYLAXIS
Yellow fever 30 (nosode): Once a week whilst travelling in endemic regions or one dose three times a week during an epidemic.

TREATMENT
Homœopathic: *Arsenicum, Belladonna, Bryonia, Carbo veg, Gelsemium, Lachesis, Phosphorus*

PART III

MATERIA MEDICA

ACONITE – ACONITUM NAPELLUS (MONKSHOOD)

Symptoms come on quickly, violently and intensely. Very useful at the beginning of a high fever or inflammation. Symptoms begin after exposure to cold or after a fright or shock. An excellent remedy for children and childhood illnesses.

Mental & Emotional:	Restless, anxious and fearful. Useful for shock following a disaster such as earthquake.
Head:	Heavy and hot. Fever with a headache. Feels bursting.
Eyes:	Conjunctivitis
Stomach:	Intense thirst. Violent vomiting.
Abdomen:	Colic. Bloody stools. Dysentery, especially on hot days.
Respiratory:	Hoarse, dry, painful cough. Croup. Laryngitis.
Fever:	Chills alternating with heat. High fever. Dry, burning heat. Drenching sweat.

MODALITIES

Worse for:	Fright, shock, night, cold.
Compare:	*Belladonna, Chamomilla, Sulphur*

APIS – APIS MELLIFICA (HONEY BEE)

Symptoms are characterised by the familiar heat, redness, burning and swelling of a bee sting. Any inflammation with heat, burning pains, redness and swelling, eg. sore throats, boils, cystitis, insect bites, may require Apis. Irritable and excitable. Everything seems wrong. Sudden shrieking.

Head:	Stabbing pains. Rolling or boring of head in pillow in meningitis. Encephalitis. Head feels swollen.
Eyes:	Conjunctivitis. Hot and red. Stinging pains.

Throat:	Swollen, red. Stinging pains on swallowing. Diphtheria with swelling and dirty membrane.
Cough:	Panting breathing. Air hunger.
Skin:	Hot swellings.

MODALITIES

Worse for:	Heat. Touch. After sleep. Insect bites and stings.
Better for:	Cool.
Compare:	*Arsenicum, Belladonna, Pulsatilla, Sulphur*

ARNICA – ARNICA MONTANA

A vital remedy for any first-aid kit. Take when there is any physical trauma or accident involving shock, bruising or bleeding. Will help to prevent shock, haemorrhage and sepsis. Take before and after any operation, childbirth or dental treatment. Useful for symptoms of over-exertion, eg. when trekking, mountaineering etc.

Mental & Emotional:	Shock. Person says there is nothing wrong when there obviously is. Fear of being touched. Coma.
Head:	Head injury.
Extremities:	Limbs feel beaten. Over exertion.
Skin:	Crops of small boils. Bruising.
Fever:	Fever following a physical trauma.

MODALITIES

Worse for:	Injury, bruises, over-exertion, labour. Touch.
Better for:	Lying down.
Compare:	*Aconite, Rhus tox*

ARSENICUM – ARSENICUM ALBUM

A very useful remedy to take when travelling. Covers many cases of diarrhoea, food poisoning, gastro-enteritis, dysentery and malaria. Symptoms are marked by anxiety and restlessness and later by prostration and weakness. Altitude sickness. Pains are often burning. Jaundice.

Mental & Emotional:	Extreme anxiety and restlessness. Fear of death. Irritable but fears being left alone. Sensitive to disorder.
Eyes:	Conjunctivitis. Intense photophobia.
Nose:	Thin, watery discharge making nose sore. Sneezing. Hayfever. Colds descending to chest.
Stomach:	Intense, burning thirst for sips of water. Vomiting and diarrhoea. Nausea with retching and vomiting. Burning pains in stomach.
Abdomen:	Diarrhoea with foul smelling, watery stools. Burning diarrhoea. Dysentery. Cholera. Swollen liver and spleen.
Cough:	Shortness of breath worse lying down, must sit up. Asthma with anxiety.
Skin:	Looks seared, dry, sore. Hives. Ulcers. Gangrene.
Fever:	Internally cold with external heat. Chills. Craves hot drinks. Intermittent fever. Chills alternating with heat. Yellow fever.

MODALITIES

Worse for:	Night or early hours of the morning. At regular intervals eg. every night, every week. Cold. Cold drinks. Bad food. Exertion.
Better for:	Hot drinks. Warmth. Sweating.
Compare:	*Aconite, Carbo veg, Lachesis, Phosphorus, Pulsatilla, Rhus tox, Sulphur, Veratrum alb*

BAPTISIA – BAPTISIA TINCTORIA (WILD INDIGO)

A remedy for septic conditions. Heaviness and aching of muscles with rapid prostration. The person looks dusky, bluish and confused. Low fever. Typhoid. Malaria. Toxaemia. Gastric influenza. Tetanus.

Mental & Emotional:	Sense of duality. Parts feel separated or scattered. Dull and confused. Hopeless of recovery. Nightmares.
Ears:	Deafness in typhoid.
Face:	Lockjaw.
Throat:	Dark, red. Spasms in throat. Cannot swallow food.
Stomach:	Sinking feeling. Gastric fever.
Abdomen:	Foul smelling sudden diarrhoea. Painless dysentery. Intestinal tox-aemia.
Cough:	Craves air.
Fever:	Lingering fever. Septic or gastric fevers.

MODALITIES

Worse for:	Humidity. Hot weather.

BELLADONNA – ATROPA BELLADONNA (DEADLY NIGHTSHADE)

Belladonna is one of the first remedies to think of where there is a high fever, especially in children. Fevers and inflammations are marked by burning heat and redness. Pains are severe and may be throbbing, cutting, shooting or like electric shocks. The symptoms tend to be of an extreme and violent nature. Sunstroke. Blood poisoning. Rabies.

Mental & Emotional:	Delirious. Noisy, cries out. Bites and strikes out. Restless. Sees monsters and fears imaginary things. Hydrophobia.
Head:	Throbbing, hammering headache. Meningitis. Rolls head. Epileptic fits.

44

Eyes:	Pupils dilated. Eyes staring. Conjunctivitis. Intense photophobia.
Ears:	Intense throbbing earache in children.
Throat:	Dry and hot. Sore. Tonsillitis.
Stomach:	Vomiting. Desires sour things and lemonade. Great thirst for cold water.
Abdomen:	Cramp and colic. Diarrhoea.
Cough:	Tickling, dry cough worse at night. Barking cough. Moaning with every breath. Whooping cough.
Extremities:	Jerks and spasms in limbs. Joints swollen, and shiny red. Trembling limbs. Cold extremities.
Skin:	Red, dry and glossy. Dry and hot. Red streaks radiating, extending up limbs. Scarlatina.
Fever:	High fever. Moans or jerks and twitches during fever. Thirstless.

MODALITIES

Worse for:	Heat of sun. Cold drafts.
Compare:	*Aconite, Arsenicum, Chamomilla, Mercurius, Sulphur*

BRYONIA – BRYONIA ALBA (WILD HOPS)

This remedy covers a wide range of symptoms especially of the mucus membranes and digestive system. Pains are usually bursting or stitching and are made worse by movement. There is a tendency to dryness. Childhood illnesses that linger or develop slowly. Influenza.

Mental & Emotional:	Very irritable. Wants to go home and be left alone.
Head:	Dizzy and faint. Splitting, heavy headache over the eyes. Hot head and red face.
Nose:	Dry and blocked. Descending colds. Sinusitis with pains around the eyes.
Throat:	Dry and sore.

Stomach:	Intense thirst for large quantities of cold water. Heaviness in the stomach. Vomiting and nausea.
Abdomen:	Liver swollen and tender. Jaundice. Constipation with large, dry hard stools. Diarrhoea in hot weather or from cold drinks. Appendicitis.
Cough:	Dry, hard and very painful cough. Holds chest when coughing. Sharp stitches in chest when breathing or coughing. Pleurisy.
Skin:	Slow development of rash in childhood illnesses. Undeveloped measles.
Fever:	Dry, burning heat. Fevers linger.
MODALITIES	
Worse for:	Motion, exertion, heat, coughing.
Better for:	Holding or lying on painful part.
Compare:	*Lycopodium, Natrum mur, Rhus tox, Sepia, Sulphur*

CALC CARB - CALCAREA CARBONICA

This is a remedy for people who tend to be overweight and flabby and who are chilly but sweat easily. Children tend to have large heads and be fearful and stubborn. It chiefly affects the glands and also the bones and skin. Adults are slow moving and children are late developers with difficult teething. They get colds easily. Defective assimilation.

Mental & Emotional	Forgetful. Melancholic. Lacks self-confidence. Fearful of disease and disaster.
Throat	Swollen glands. Tonsilitis.
Abdomen	Swollen. Distended. Gall-stone colic. Flatulence. Glands swollen and painful. Colic. Children's diarrhoea. Chronic diarrhoea or dysentery.
Cough	Habitual cough. Short of breath.
MODALITIES	
Worse for:	Cold. Exertion. Teething. Milk.

CAMPHOR – CAMPHORA

Camphor is one of the classic remedies in the treatment of cholera. The key symptoms are an icy coldness of the skin combined with a sudden and total collapse of the patient.

Stomach:	Extreme thirst. Burning pain.
Abdomen:	Colourless 'rice water' stools. Cholera. Absent stool with collapse.
Fever:	Chill with cold skin but doesn't want covers. Sudden fever with rapid prostration.
Compare:	*Carbo veg, Cuprum, Opium, Veratrum alb*

CARBO VEG – CARBO VEGETABILIS

A life saving remedy for people who are not recovering from an illness. The vitality may become very low during an acute illness or sudden collapse may occur. The patient becomes almost lifeless, with a cold body, cold breath, faint pulse and quickened respiration. The person may look pinched, blue or very pale. Useful for old people. Lack of reaction. Cholera. Typhoid.

Head:	Dull, heavy headache. Cold sweat on forehead. Head may be hot when rest of body is cold.
Stomach:	All food turns to gas. Averse to all food. Nausea. Loud, rancid or painful eructations. Heaviness in stomach. Gastralgia. Vomiting of blood.
Abdomen:	Excessive flatulence. Distended abdomen. Colic. Painful liver. Painful, putrid diarrhoea with much urging. Jaundice.
Cough:	Air hunger. Complications of whooping cough. Breathing laborious.
Fever:	Icy coldness. Internal burning heat. Alternate chill and heat. Yellow fever.
Compare:	*Arsenicum, China, Lachesis, Phosphorus*

CHAMOMILLA – MATRICARIA CHAMOMILLA (GERMAN CHAMOMILE)

Chamomilla is one of the most important children's remedies. Try this if the infant or child is crying as if in pain but there are no other symptoms. The symptoms are marked by irritability, and restlessness and that any pain is experienced as unbearable and agonising. Symptoms may come on in teething children.

Mental & Emotional:	Cross and irritable. Children want to be carried and scream if put down. Wants things that are refused when offered.
Ear:	Earache very painful in children.
Face:	One cheek red.
Stomach:	Violent retching and vomiting. Bitter vomit.
Abdomen:	Colic worse at night. Diarrhoea. Stools green, yellow, slimy or smelling like bad eggs. Jaundice.
Cough:	Dry, tickling cough. Whooping cough. Anger provokes the cough.
Fever:	Alternate chill and heat. Chill of one part with heat in another. Thirst during fever

MODALITIES

Worse for:	Anger. Night. Teething. Cold.
Better for:	Being carried. Warmth. Sweating.
Compare:	*Aconite, Belladonna, Nux vomica, Pulsatilla*

CHINA – CHINA OFFICINALIS (QUININE)

China is a key remedy for profuse and exhausting discharges, eg diarrhoea, haemorrhage, etc. It affects the blood and circulation with symptoms of weakness, haemorrhage and anaemia. It is an important remedy for sepsis, tropical fevers and malaria. China has been used as an alternative to blood transfusions following haemorrhage or blood loss.

Mental & Emotional:	Weakness, oversensitivity and nervousness. Indifference. Daydreaming.
Stomach:	Loud belching without relief. Frequent vomiting. Hungry and yet averse to any food.
Abdomen:	Liver and spleen enlarged. Flatulence and bloating. Colic. Post operative gas pains. Jaundice. Dark, foul, watery or bloody stools. Painless diarrhoea. Chronic diarrhoea.
Cough:	Rattling breathing. Painfully sore chest. Coughs up blood.
Fever:	Stages of chill, then heat then sweat well marked. Hectic fever. Drenching, exhausting sweats worse at night.

MODALITIES

Worse for:	Loss of bodily fluids. Touch. Cold. Bad food or water. Fruit.
Compare:	*Carbo veg*

COCCUS CACTI (COCHINEAL)

A remedy for spasmodic or whooping coughs especially when associated with profuse, thick, clear mucous.

Throat:	Accumulation of mucous with hawking and scraping. Clearing throat excites the cough. Tickling in throat. Profuse post-nasal catarrh.
Cough:	Fits of paroxysmal, violent cough. Cough ends in vomiting of food or thick stringy mucous. Clear mucous hangs from mouth. Face goes purple or red during coughing fit. Cough builds up slowly and then decreases slowly.
Fever:	Burning heat.

MODALITIES

Worse for:	Heat. Lying down. At regular intervals.

Better for:	Cold drinks
Compare:	*Drosera, Phosphorus*

CUPRUM – CUPRUM METALLICUM (COPPER)

Cuprum affects the nerves and muscles causing spasms, convulsions and cramps. The face may have a blue or sunken look. It is a key remedy for cholera when there are excessive cramps, not only in the abdomen, but also in the fingers and toes. Tetanus.

Mental & Emotional:	Confusion. Piercing shrieks.
Head:	Vertigo. Epileptic fits. Meningitis.
Face:	Blue, pinched, sunken. Lockjaw.
Stomach:	Vomiting with agonising colic. Vomits on least motion. Foecal vomiting.
Abdomen:	Agonising colic with contraction of the abdomen. Abdomen tense, contracted, prone to spasm. Diarrhoea profuse, spurts out. Green, watery stools. Cholera. Summer diarrhoea.
Cough:	Violent, paroxysmal. Cough alternates with spasmodic vomiting. Whooping cough. Shortness of breath. Rattling in chest.
Extremities:	Cramps in hands, calves and feet. Jerking limbs. Joints and muscles contracted.
Fever:	Icy coldness of skin. Cold, clammy sweat.
Compare:	*Veratrum alb*

DROSERA – DROSERA ROTUNDIFOLIA (SUNDEW)

A classic remedy for whooping cough.

Mental & Emotional: Very irritable.

Eyes:	Become prominent with a cough or during measles.
Cough:	Cough is barking, choking, prolonged and incessant. It comes from the abdomen and takes the breath away. Person holds their sides when coughing. Cough followed by retching and vomiting of food or mucous. Nose bleed with cough. Deep hoarse voice. Tickling in throat. Cough comes on after measles.
Fever:	Fever with whooping cough. Chilly.

MODALITIES

Worse for:	At night. Lying down.
Compare:	*Coccus cacti, Sulphur*

EUPATORIUM – EUPATORIUM PERFOLIATUM (BONESET)

Characterised by violent aching pains in the muscles and bones. Muscles, back, chest and limbs can all feel bruised, sore and aching. Influenza. Malaria.

Head:	Throbbing. Vertigo. Soreness of eyeballs.
Stomach:	Nausea at sight of food. Bilious vomiting.
Cough:	Sore chest and bronchi. Holds chest when coughing.
Fever:	Violent shaking chill. Severe bone pains before fever.
Compare:	*Bryonia, Gelsemium*

EUPHRASIA (EYEBRIGHT)

A remedy for inflamed mucus membranes especially eyes. Colds. Hayfever. Measles.

Head:	Catarrhal headache.
Eyes:	Watery eyes. Eyes feel hot and sore. Photophobia. Conjunctivitis.
Nose:	Profuse runny nose.
Cough:	Cough worse in day time.
Compare:	*Arsenicum, Pulsatilla*

FERRUM PHOS – FERRUM PHOSPHORICUM

This is one of the Biochemic Tissue Salts and is useful for a wide range of feverish and inflammatory conditions. Take at the beginning of any fever, cough, inflammation etc. and it may prevent any further symptoms developing. Anaemia. Measles. Childhood diseases.

Head:	Throbbing headache. Sunstroke. Toothache.
Ears:	Violent earache.
Nose:	Nosebleeds especially in children.
Throat:	Sore inflamed throat. Hoarseness.
Abdomen:	Bloody and watery stools. Dysentery with fever. Summer diarrhoea.
Cough:	Laryngitis. Tickling cough.
Fever:	Initial stages of all fevers.

GELSEMIUM (YELLOW JASMINE)

An important remedy where illness causes weakness, trembling and aching. Weakness and paralysis of muscles. Aching, tiredness and heaviness in the limbs. A classic influenza remedy. Polio.

Mental & Emotional:	Anxiety and trembling before an ordeal eg. exams, flying etc. Drowsiness. Confusion. Coma.
Head:	Vertigo. Dull, heavy or band-like headache. Meningitis.

Eyes:	Heavy, drooping eyelids. Shaking vision. Aching.
Throat:	Swallowing difficult. Paralysis.
Abdomen:	Diarrhoea. Paralysis of anus. Diarrhoea after emotional trauma.
Extremities:	Knees weak. Aching. Cramps. Paralysis.
Fever:	Chills with aching alternating with heat. Chills up and down back. Thirst absent.

MODALITIES

Worse for:	Emotional ordeals. Humid weather. Spring.
Better for:	Urinating. Sweating. Alcoholic drinks.
Compare:	*Eupatorium*

HYPERICUM – HYPERICUM PERFORATUM (ST JOHN'S WORT)

An excellent first-aid remedy to give following injury to a part of the body rich in nerve endings, eg. fingers, toes or spinal cord. The injury will be very painful because the nerves have been damaged. Pains will be shooting, burning or throbbing. Punctured or lacerated wounds. Cases of tetanus, particularly after the onset; give Ledum initially and Hypericum if any symptoms develop. Spinal injury or where limbs are crushed. Jerking and spasms in limbs. Post-operative pains. Painful burns. Sepsis. Boils.

MODALITIES

Worse for:	Injury, jar, concussion, shock, touch, motion.
Compare:	*Arnica, Ledum*

IPECAC – IPECACUANA

This remedy acts on the pneumo-gastric nerve and produces mainly symptoms of the digestive system and the respiratory system. It is well known as a remedy for nausea and also for asthma and whooping cough. There is also a tendency to haemorrhage.

Head:	Headache with nausea and vomiting.
Stomach:	Horrible nausea not relieved by vomiting. Nausea with a clean tongue. Morning sickness of pregnancy.
Abdomen:	Cutting pains. Brown or bloody diarrhoea. Dysentery with nausea.
Cough:	Gasps for breath. Asthma. Incessant, violent, paroxysmal cough. Suffocative cough with retching. Whooping cough; child stiffens out, their face becomes red or blue and then they gag and vomit. Bloody expectoration. Rattling in chest without expectoration.
Fever:	Fever with nausea. Short chill then long heat. Gastric influenza.
Compare:	*Ant tart, Coccus cacti, Drosera*

LAC CANINUM (DOG'S MILK)

Chiefly affects the glands of the throat and the breasts. Symptoms alternate from side to side. Person is very sensitive to touch. Diphtheria. Mumps. Dries up breast milk when weaning.

Mental & Emotional:	Full of imaginings. Dreams of snakes.
Throat:	Sore, red and glistening. Milky, white membrane in diphtheria. Symptoms eg. swelling change repeatedly from side to side. Swallowing difficult, pain extends to the ears.

MODALITIES

Worse for:	Touch, during menses, cold air.
Compare:	*Lachesis, Phytolacca, Pulsatilla*

LACHESIS (BUSHMASTER SNAKE)

Lachesis decomposes the blood causing a tendency to haemorrhage and sepsis. The circulation is affected with parts becoming hot or blue. People needing this remedy hate anything tight on their body and dislike warmth. Symptoms often begin on the left side and then move to the right side, eg. mumps. Their symptoms are worse on waking up. The throat is very much affected. Diphtheria and carriers of diphtheria. Gangrene.

Mental & Emotional:	Talkative. Jealous. Suspicious. Delusions.
Throat:	Sensation of a lump in the throat. Septic mumps. Swallowing painful. Throat pains extend to the ear.
Cough:	Sensation of suffocation.
Skin:	Mottled, bluish or purple. Ulcers.
Fever:	Flushes of heat. Feet icy cold.

MODALITIES

Worse for:	After sleep, mornings, heat, spring, sun, swallowing, pressure of clothes especially around waist or neck, alcohol.
Better for:	Open air, free discharges, cold drinks.
Compare:	*Lycopodium, Sepia, Sulphur*

LATHYRUS (CHICK-PEA)

A remedy for effects of the lateral and anterior columns of the spinal cord with paralysis of the lower limbs. Wasting diseases with weakness and heaviness. Slow recovery of nerve power. Spastic paralysis. Infantile paralysis. Poliomyelitis.

Extremities:	Paralysis. Stiffness and lameness. Reflexes are increased. Lower limbs emaciated. Muscles of calves very tense. Spasms.

LEDUM – LEDUM PALUSTRE (MARSH TEA)

An excellent first-aid remedy for punctured wounds caused by rusty nails, wire, thorns, animal bites, insect stings, splinters, etc. It will help prevent sepsis and if given quickly enough will be effective against tetanus. Also good for bruising with much blackness and puffiness eg. black eye. Pains are sticking, pricking and throbbing. The skin may feel cold to the touch but the person dislikes heat. Swelling with localised twitching. Wasp stings.

MODALITIES

Worse for:	Warmth, punctured wounds, injury.
Better for:	Cold bathing.
Compare:	*Arnica, Hypericum*

LYCOPODIUM – LYCOPODIUM CLAVATUM (CLUB MOSS)

A remedy marked by weakness of the digestion and a disturbed liver. There will be symptoms of gas and acidity. Symptoms tend to be right sided or move from right to left. Highly developed intellectually but physically weak and fearful.

Mental & Emotional:	Mentally active but growing weak physically. Confusion. Fearful of being alone.
Head:	Deep furrows on forehead.
Nose:	Fan like motion of nostrils with lung or digestive system diseases.
Stomach:	Weak digestion. Eating a tiny amount causes fullness. Bilious vomiting.
Abdomen:	Bloated. Noisy flatulence better passing wind. Chronic hepatitis.
Cough:	Dry, tickling chronic cough. Cough with emaciation. Craves air. Neglected pneumonia.
Fever:	Coldness and chills.

MODALITIES

Worse for:	Warm room, 4 to 8pm.
Better for:	Warm drinks. Eructations.
Compare:	*Carbo veg, Pulsatilla, Sulphur*

MERCURIUS – MERCURIUS SOLUBILIS (MERCURY)

A remedy with marked affects on the glands. Lymphatic, salivary and mucous glands may all be enlarged. There tends to be an increase in secretions and discharges eg. saliva, mucous, urine, sweat, etc. There also tends to be an offensiveness in the symptoms, eg. bad breath, smelly diarrhoea. There may also be weakness and trembling. Mumps. Measles.

Mental & Emotional:	Stammering, nervous. Violent impulses.
Head:	Vertigo with swinging sensation. Band feeling about the head. Meningitis.
Ears:	Earache with sharp pains worse at night. Yellow discharge. Measles affecting the ears.
Nose:	Much sneezing. Acrid discharge. Sore, swollen nose. Colds travel to eyes.
Mouth:	Excessive saliva. Gums spongy and bleeding. Horribly bad breath. Tongue flabby, coated and indented. Metallic taste.
Throat:	Sore, raw throat. Tonsilitis. Stitching pain extends to ears on swallowing. Ulcers in mouth or throat.
Abdomen:	Liver enlarged and sore. Greenish or bloody diarrhoea with much mucous and a foul smell. Dysentery. Never get done feeling with diarrhoea.
Skin:	Ulcers. Moist, crusty eruptions. Moist eczema.

Fever:	Easily chilled or overheated. Profuse sweat especially at night.
MODALITIES	
Worse for:	Night, sweating, heat, changing weather, extremes of temperature.
Compare:	*Belladonna, Lachesis, Phytolacca, Sulphur*

NATRUM MUR – NATRUM MURIATICUM (COMMON SALT)

An important homœopathic remedy with marked mental and physical symptoms. People needing this remedy tend to be serious and reserved and they dislike fuss or consolation. The symptoms may come on after grief or disappointment. There are often symptoms of dryness and weakness. A useful remedy for prolonged malaria or where the person has never really recovered from malaria. Colds.

Mental & Emotional:	Depressed especially following grief, disappointment, etc. Consolation aggravates. Irritable. Wants to be alone to cry.
Head:	Headache hammering over the eyes. Headaches with disturbed vision.
Eyes:	Watering eyes.
Nose:	Colds with alternating runny and then stuffed up nose.
Face:	Herpetic eruptions on lips or nose.
Abdomen:	Constipation with dry, hard stools.
Skin:	Greasy skin. Herpes.
Fever:	Heat with thirst. Prolonged chills. Periodic fever. Chronic malaria.
MODALITIES	
Worse for:	Mornings, heat of sun, sympathy, sea-side.
Better for:	Open air, sweating, missing meals.
Compare:	*Bryonia, Pulsatilla, Sepia*

NATRUM SULPH – NATRUM SULPHURICUM (GLAUBER'S SALT)

A liver remedy especially where symptoms are worse in damp, humid or wet weather. Discharges are often yellow.

Mental & Emotional: Sensitive and suspicious. Mental troubles following an injury to the head.

Head: Useful to give following any injury to the head. Spinal meningitis.

Stomach: Green bilious vomiting. Acidity. Nausea.

Abdomen: Liver region sore and tender. Hepatitis. Painful flatulence. Rumbling and gurgling in bowels followed by sudden, noisy and spluttering stools. Morning diarrhoea. Dysentery. Giardia. Yellow diarrhoea.

Cough: Asthma worse damp weather and worse exertion. Loose, violent cough. Shortness of breath.

MODALITIES

Worse for: Damp, damp cellars or basements, lying on left side, head injuries.

Better for: Warm dry air.

Compare: *Arsenicum, Pulsatilla*

NUX VOMICA (POISON NUT)

An important remedy for a wide range of symptoms arising chiefly from overdoing things. Appropriate for forceful people who push themselves hard. Also useful for symptoms coming on after overindulgence in food and drink eg. hangovers. A wide range of digestive disorders.

Mental & Emotional: Very irritable. Over sensitive. Aggressive and impatient. Ill effects of prolonged mental work eg. studying, business, etc.

Head: Headache from overindulgence of alcohol. Vertigo worse when hungry.

Nose:	Violent sneezing. Runny nose or running of one nostril only.
Stomach:	Hiccoughs. Sour or bitter vomiting. Heartburn. Eructations. Nausea greatly relieved by vomiting. Violent vomiting. Food lies heavy in the stomach. Indigestion from spicy or rich food.
Abdomen:	Bruised, sore feeling. Cannot bear anything tight round waist. Constipation with fitful and fruitless urging. Diarrhoea with jaundice. Dysentery when person feels better for a little while after every bout of diarrhoea. Painful, itching haemorrhoids.
Cough:	Violent, paroxysmal cough. Cough causes headache. Whooping cough.
Fever:	Extreme chill, cannot uncover. Skin hot but person easily chilled.

MODALITIES

Worse for:	Early morning, mental exertion, cold, uncovering, high living, spicy food, stimulants, drugs, anger, pressure of clothes.
Better for:	Sleep, rest, free discharges, moist air.
Compare:	*Arsenicum, Lycopodium, Phosphorus, Sulphur*

PHOSPHORUS

An element which causes degeneration of the mucus membranes, nerves and blood vessels. Great tendency to haemorrhage. Diseases which worsen becoming debilitating and of a destructive nature. Burning pains. Liver diseases. Osteomyelitis.

Mental & Emotional: Liveliness followed by exhaustion. Excitable. Fearful, sees things creeping out of the corner. Fears dark, ghosts, the future.

Nose:	Fan like motion of nostrils. Nosebleeds. Sneezing and coryza. Descending nose colds.
Stomach:	Craves cold drinks which are vomited after a short time. Nausea following general anaesthetic. Regurgitates ingesta. Ravenous hunger followed by vomiting. Vomits bile or blood. Burning pains. Empty feeling.
Abdomen:	Stools slender or watery and foetid. Exhausting diarrhoea. Dysentery. Acute hepatitis. Malignant jaundice. Atrophy of liver. Anal haemorrhage.
Respiratory:	Tightness of chest. Raw, sore larynx with a husky voice. Bronchitis. Tickling, painful hacking cough. Copious expectoration. Haemorrhage of lungs. Pneumonia.
Extremities:	Paralysis moves inwards from fingers and toes. Pins and needles. Burning pains. Cramps. Weakness and trembling of limbs. Post-diphtheriatic paralysis.
Fever:	Craves ice. Burning heat. Hectic. Painless fevers.

MODALITIES

Worse for:	Emotions, cold, warm ingesta, sexual excess, sudden change in weather, twilight, exhaustion.
Better for:	Sleep, eating, cold food, rubbing.
Compare:	*Arsenicum, Lycopodium, Nux vomica, Pulsatilla*

PHYTOLACCA (POKE ROOT)

Primarily a glandular remedy. Glandular swellings with heat and inflammation. Sore throat, tonsillitis, mumps and diphtheria. Mastitis. Affected parts become bluish-red. Symptoms cause soreness and aching.

Throat:	Dark or bluish red. Sore, dry throat very painful on swallowing. Feels as if a lump in the throat. Cannot swallow anything hot. White or grey spots. Shooting pain into the ears on swallowing. Throat feels very hot. Pain at root of tongue.

MODALITIES

Worse for:	Getting up, motion, swallowing, hot drinks.
Better for:	Rest.
Compare:	*Bryonia, Lachesis, Mercurius, Pulsatilla*

PULSATILLA (WIND FLOWER)

An important homœopathic remedy especially for children. Mental symptoms are often marked. Other symptoms are often of the glands and digestion. Childhood illnesses: measles, mumps.

Mental & Emotional:	Someone needing this remedy when ill will become mild, emotional and weepy. Children become tearful, whiny and clingy, wanting lots of fuss, comforting and attention. Fearful and timid.
Eyes:	Thick, yellow bland discharge. Conjunctivitis from colds. Itching eyes. Hayfever. Watering eyes.
Ears:	Earache worse at night. Catarrhal deafness, as if ears stopped up. Discharge of pus or blood. Swollen.
Nose:	Stuffed up, better in the open air. Green or yellow nasal discharge.
Mouth:	Dry mouth but no thirst. Bad taste in mouth.
Throat:	Feels swollen, dry. Mumps. Metastases of mumps to testes or to breasts and ovaries.

Stomach:	Indigestion from fats, pork or pastries. Thirstless. Stomach feels heavy, weighed down as from a stone. Vomiting with nausea and heartburn. Averse fatty food.
Abdomen:	Diarrhoea. Stools are changeable.
Cough:	Shortness of breath. Cough loose in the morning, dry at night. Must sit up in bed when coughing. Heaviness of chest. Cough after measles.
Skin:	Itching worse when heated. Urticaria. Measles rash.
Fever:	Chilly yet craves open, fresh air. Cold even in warm room. Feverish.

MODALITIES

Worse for:	Warmth, evening, rest, after eating, rich foods, puberty, pregnancy, before menses.
Better for:	Fresh air, sitting erect, after a good cry.
Compare:	*Arsenicum, Natrum mur, Sepia*

PYROGEN – PYROGENIUM (ARTIFICIAL SEPSIN)

A great remedy for septic states. Septic fevers. All discharges are horribly offensive. Restlessness is very marked, there also tend to be bruised, aching and sore pains. Hectic fevers, typhoid, typhus, poisonings, septic wounds, diphtheria, chronic malaria, after-effects of operations and miscarriage. Heart failure threatens from septic state.

Mental & Emotional:	Talkative. Sensitive, anxious, confused. Sense of duality; of too many arms and legs.
Mouth:	Horribly offensive breath.
Stomach:	Persistent vomiting. Vomiting: coffee grounds, faecal, offensive. Great thirst especially for cold drinks but any liquid is instantly vomited.

Abdomen:	Horribly offensive stools. Brown or black painless stools. Constipation.
Extremities:	Aching in all limbs and bones.
Skin:	Offensive ulcers. Any cut or injury becomes very swollen and inflamed. Rosy red streaks, lymphangitis. Abscesses with pain and burning.
Fever:	Chills, felt in bones. Hectic. Quickly oscillating temperature. Pulse rapid, out of proportion to temperature.

MODALITIES

Worse for:	Cold, damp, motion
Better for:	Heat, pressure, changing position
Compare:	*Arsenicum, Baptisia, Belladonna, Lachesis*

RHUS TOX – RHUS TOXICODENDRON (POISON IVY)

This is an effective remedy for irritations of the skin and for rheumatic symptoms. It is also a remedy for certain types of fever including influenza, measles and typhoid like fevers. The symptoms are often painful with either tearing, shooting and stitching pains or sore, bruised and aching pains. Symptoms often come on after getting cold and wet. The person tends to be restless.

Mental & Emotional:	Anxious, sad and restless. Confusion. Exhausting dreams.
Eyes:	Pain behind eyes. Sticky eyelids. Inflamed. Paralysis of muscles of eyeball.
Tongue:	Triangular red tip.
Throat:	Sore throat with swollen glands. Throat red and puffy, difficulty swallowing.
Abdomen:	Sore. Ileo-caecal symptoms; appendicitis. Stools are watery, frothy, bloody,

	slimy or like meat water. Painful urging without stool.
Cough:	Dry, hoarse, tormenting.
Extremities:	Numbness and pins and needles. Limbs stiff or paralysed. Rheumatic aching worse after resting, eased when gently moving or walking; also much worse on beginning to move. Hot painful swelling of joints. Pulled or torn muscles. Cramps in calves.
Skin:	Intense itching. Moist, crusty eruptions. Measles rash. Rash worse on hairy parts of the body. Urticaria. Shingles. Chicken pox.
Fever:	Easily chilled, likes to be covered. Aching in limbs during fever. Restless delirium. Chill in single parts. Typhoid.

MODALITIES

Worse for:	Exposure to cold wet weather, rest, sprains, over-exertion, cold drinks, after midnight.
Better for:	Gentle continued motion, heat, hot bath, rubbing, change of position.
Compare:	*Arsenicum, Bryonia, Phytolacca*

SEPIA (INKY JUICE OF CUTTLEFISH)

A remedy with many symptoms of stagnancy, congestion and weakness. It is often used for complaints that come on during pregnancy. The person may look yellowish.

Mental & Emotional: The person complains of weariness and hopelessness. Indifference especially to family and loved ones. Anxious about health and family. Indifference alternating with irritability. Feels better when physically or mentally active or sociable but exhausted afterwards.

Head:	Headache with shooting pains or heavy and accompanied with nausea. Headache with jaundice.
Face:	Drooping eyelids. Dark circles under eyes. Brown or yellowish stripe across nose.
Stomach:	Nausea especially at thought or smell of food. Morning sickness. Faint, sinking feeling in the stomach. Sudden hunger. Sour risings. Foul taste in mouth.
Abdomen:	Heavy, bearing down feeling. Liver sore and painful. Pot-bellied. Obstinate constipation. Diarrhoea with exhaustion. Haemorrhoids. Jelly-like, offensive mucous from bowels.
Respiratory:	Dry, fatiguing cough. Shortness of breath. Neglected pneumonia. Whooping cough that drags on causing weakness.
Skin:	Itching vesicles. Ringworm. Rough, hard cracked skin.
Fever:	Easily chilled. Cold in spots. Anxious hot flushes. Easy, offensive sweat.

MODALITIES

Worse for:	Cold, pregnancy, miscarriage, coition
Better for:	Violent motion, warmth
Compare:	*Lachesis, Natrum mur, Nux vom, Phosphorus, Pulsatilla, Sulphur*

SULPHUR

An important homœopathic remedy that covers a wide range of symptoms. The main effects are on the skin and digestive system. A major remedy for diarrhoea and dysentery, if you are unsure of a remedy then try this one first. There is often a sensation of heat and symptoms tend to be worse when hot. It is useful for any complaint that drags on without responding to treatment or that relapses after appearing to improve.

Mental & Emotional: Irritable, critical and nagging or apathetic and depressed. Lazy. Daydreamers. Inclined to mental but not physical activity. Thinking becomes difficult.

Head: Top of head is hot or throbbing and sore. Headache with vomiting.

Nose: Fluent, burning coryza.

Stomach: Eats little but drinks a lot. Ravenous hunger but cannot eat. Sudden weakness and hunger, especially at 11am. Eructations. Sour vomiting with heaviness in stomach. Acidity. Milk disagrees. Useful for people who have over-indulged for years in over-eating and alcohol.

Abdomen: Pain and soreness over liver. Very sensitive to pressure. Itching, painful haemorrhoids. Chronic or relapsing jaundice. Hepatitis. Stitches in liver. Diarrhoea with rushing to toilet, worse early in the morning. Stools foul smelling, painless and watery. Diarrhoea in infants. Dysentery.

Cough: Shortness of breath, difficult breathing. Craves fresh air. Violent cough in incomplete bouts. Rattling of mucous in chest. Shooting pains or heat in chest. Neglected pneumonia.

Skin: Many kinds of rash and eruptions are covered by this remedy. Itching is very marked, which is worse at night, in bed and when warm. Wounds fester and are slow to heal. Eruptions alternate with other complaints.

Fever: Flushes of heat. Profuse sweat. Remittent fever. Malaria.

MODALITIES

Worse for:	Suppressions, bathing, milk, warmth, over-exertion, in bed
Compare:	*Arsenicum, Bryonia, Lachesis, Lycopodium, Nux vomica, Rhus tox, Sepia*

VERATRUM ALB – VERATRUM ALBUM (WHITE HELLEBORE)

A remedy marked by copious evacuations and rapid prostration. Coldness and collapse are rapid. Cholera with cold sweats.

Face:	Cold sweat on forehead. Bluish, pale.
Stomach:	Excessive vomiting with purging. Violent retching. Craves ice-cold water, fruit and cold food.
Abdomen:	Cutting colic with cramps in limbs. Watery, green or colourless (rice water) stools. Straining for stool until exhausted. Peritonitis.
Cough:	Continuous violent cough with retching. Loss of voice. Neglected whooping cough.
Extremities:	Cramps in calves during stools.
Fever:	Cold sweat. Icy coldness of parts. Internal heat with cold skin.

MODALITIES

Worse for:	Drinking cold drinks when warm, fruit, exertion.
Compare:	*Arsenicum, Camphor, Carbo veg, Cuprum*

APPENDICES

TRAVEL/FIRST-AID KIT

These are the remedies that I always keep handy in the home and take with me when travelling.

OINTMENTS

Arnica: For bruising, injury, sprains & strains etc. Apply directly to the injured part, but do not use on broken skin.

Hypercal: (*Hypericum* and *Calendula* combined). An excellent general purpose antiseptic and healing ointment. Use on abrasions, cuts, spots, insect bites, etc.

Burn Cream: Most homœopathic pharmacies stock a burn cream, usually based on a combination of *Urtica* and *Hypericum* with other tinctures added. Use on minor burns and scalds and sunburn.

TINCTURES

Hypercal: (*Hypericum* and *Calendula* combined). An antiseptic and healing lotion, will prevent wounds going septic. Apply neat for small cuts, insect bites, spots, etc. To clean wounds dilute a few drops in a little cool, boiled water and gently bathe the area using a piece of cotton wool dipped in the solution.

Pyrethrum: This can be bought as a spray from many homœopathic pharmacies to use as a first-aid treatment for insect bites and stings.

HERBS

Chamomile: Take a few of these teabags with you. Take as an infusion for any feverish conditions, spasmodic pains such as period pains, indigestion and also insomnia or stress. Safe to give to infants. Externally use the infusion as a soothing wash for inflammation or itching rashes etc. Use the cooled infusion as an eyewash for eye infections, sore eyes, etc.

ESSENTIAL OILS

Citronella: A mosquito repellent that can be diluted and applied to the skin or burnt in a room.

Lavender: Antiseptic and anti-inflammatory. Pour neat onto minor burns and scalds. Hold near the nose and inhale the vapours if feeling faint. Add a few drops to a bath for stress or insomnia. Massage a little onto the temples to relieve a headache.

Tea Tree: Antiseptic and antiviral. Pour neat onto wounds, cuts, etc. It will not sting and helps to prevent infection. Use as a steam inhalation for colds, flu and chest infections. Use as a bath or compress for fungal infections of the skin.

BACH FLOWER REMEDIES

Rescue Remedy: For shock, fear and panic. Can be taken as often as needed if involved in any accident or trauma, emotional or physical. Also good for fear eg. of flying, stagefright, etc. Take a few drops straight in the mouth or add a few drops to a little water and sip as often as required.

71

HOMŒOPATHIC REMEDIES

The following ten remedies form the basis for a first-aid kit. For indications beyond those given, look them up in the Materia Medica section of this book. Other remedies should be added according to your individual needs.

Aconite 30:	First stages of fever and inflammation; after-effects of exposure to a cold wind; earache; hoarse, dry cough; after-effects of shock or fright.
Arnica 30:	A vital part of any first-aid kit. Take following any accident or injury. Helps to reduce bruising, prevent haemorrhage, and ameliorate shock; concussion; over-exertion.
Arsenicum 30:	Food poisoning. After-effects of bad food or drink with diarrhoea and vomiting; exhaustion, anxiety and restlessness. Acute asthmatic and allergy attacks marked by anxiety. Worse at night.
Belladonna 200:	Fevers with a high temperature. Patient is hot, red and may be delirious. Sunstroke. Blood poisoning or inflammation where the affected part looks red and has a violent throbbing pain. Throbbing, hammering headache.
Ferrum phos 6X:	For the beginning stages of a cold, fever or sore throat; hoarseness; nosebleeds. Externally this remedy may be used by crushing a tablet and sprinkling the powder onto a wound to stop the bleeding and help prevent infection.
Gelsemium 30:	Influenza with an aching body, heavy headache and shivery feeling. Trembling and diarrhoea before an ordeal, or following a shock.

Hypericum 30:	Injury to parts rich in nerves, such as fingers or spine. Any injury marked by severe pain. Will heal lacerated or punctured wounds and painful burns. Festering insect bites.
Ledum 30:	Wasp, bee or other insect bites or stings. Animal bites, such as dog bites with bruising surrounding the wound. Bruising. Prophylactic for tetanus.
Nux vomica 30:	Indigestion. After-effects of over-indulgence in food, drink or stimulants (hangover). Any stomach disorder where there is nausea that is greatly relieved for a while by vomiting.
Rhus tox 30:	Sprains and strains following an injury or over-exertion. The painful or injured part swells or stiffens up during rest, and is ameliorated by gentle motion. Colds or flu following exposure to cold, wet weather. Poison ivy rash.

NOTES FOR TRAVELLERS

There are some basic steps to take that will help you stay healthy when travelling.

Firstly, preparation:
Research into the areas that you will be visiting, then consult the relevant disease sections of this book and take the appropriate remedies with you. Information about which diseases are prevalent in which areas is available from larger tour operators and larger NHS Health Centres (GP practices).

Some things to consider taking with you:
A basic travel/first-aid kit (see previous Appendix)
A supply of sterile dressings
A one-cup sized electric element for boiling water to drink, brush teeth, etc. Available from camping shops.

Finally, some things to avoid:
Avoid drinking or cleaning your teeth in contaminated water
Avoid eating doubtful foods
Avoid swimming in contaminated water
Avoid being bitten

NOTES FOR PARENTS

Many health care professionals will put pressure on you to vaccinate your child starting soon after the birth. If you have chosen not to do so then be prepared with your facts before appointments with Health Visitors, Doctors, etc. There is no legal requirement for you to have your child vaccinated in the UK.

If you have not made up your mind about immunisation, or you want to prepare yourself for discussions with your Doctor, etc, then talk to your homœopath and/or use some of the books from the reading list. The booklet, "Mass Immunisation" by Trevor Gunn is probably the most accessible.

It is also advisable to do the following:
Make contact with a practitioner you trust before your child becomes ill, (see the list of Contacts in the Appendix)
Keep a stock of basic homœopathic remedies in the house and when travelling, (see previous Appendix)

USEFUL CONTACTS AND SUPPLIERS

HOMŒOPATHY

Society of Homœopaths
2 Artizan Road
Northampton NN1 4HU
(01604) 621400
Send A5 sae for regional list of
registered homœopaths

MEDICAL HERBALISM

National Institute of Medical
Herbalists
56 Longbrook St
Exeter EX4 6ΛH
(01392) 426022
Send sae for regional list of
registered members

VACCINATION, UK

The Informed Parent
PO Box 870
Harrow
Middlesex HA3 7UW
0181-861 1022
Publish regular newsletters and
provide information

What Doctors Don't Tell You
4 Wallace Road
London N1 2PG
Publish a monthly newsletter,
pamphlets and organise talks.

Vaccination Awareness Network
178 Mansfield Road
Nottingham NG1 3HW
0115 948 0829
E-mail: info@vanuk.force9.co.uk
Web: www.vanuk.force9.co.uk
Support group, meetings and
newsletter

JABS
1 Gawsworth Road
Golborne
Warrington WA3 3RF
Tel: 01942 713565
Information and support for
parents who suspect their child
may be vaccine damaged.

VACCINATION, USA

The National Health Federation
212 W Foothill Blvd
POBox 688
Monrovia
CA 91016
Information about vaccination
and how to avoid it

Dissatisfied Parents Together
(DPT)
128 Branch Road
Vienna
VA22180
Tel: 703 938 DPT3
Information and support for
parents who suspect their
children may be vaccine dam-
aged.

CHILDHOOD ILLNESSES CONTACT NETWORK, UK

If you want your child to have the opportunity to get the common childhood illnesses, the following voluntary contacts coordinate phone arounds when there is a case of Measles, Mumps, Rubella or Chicken Pox in your area. Simply write or phone and ask to be placed on their list.

England
Lesley Dove
4 Wooster Mews
Harrow
Middlesex HA2 6QS
0181-861 1233

Wales, Hereford and
Worcestershire
Gail Venables
1 Hall Lane
New Radnor
Presteigne
Powys LD8 2SW

SUPPLIERS, UK

Neal's Yard Remedies
15 Neal's Yard
Covent Garden
London WC2H 9DP
(0171) 379 7222
Mail Order (0161) 831 7875
Suppliers of medicinal herbs and tinctures, essential oils, books and homœopathic remedies through regional shops and mail order.
For other shop addresses:
phone 0171 627 1949
or e-mail:
mail@nealsyardremedies.com

Helios Homœopathic Pharmacy
97 Camden Road
Tunbridge Wells
Kent TN1 2QR
(01892) 536393/537254
Web: www.helios.co.uk
e-mail: pharmacy@helios.co.uk
Postal service available

Ainsworths Homœopathic
Pharmacy
36 New Cavendish Street
London W1M 7LH
(0171) 935 5330
Fax 0171 627 1949
Web: Ainsworths.com
e-mail: ainshome@msn.com
Postal service available

SUGGESTED READING

VACCINATION

Allen, H., *Don't Get Stuck! The Case Against Vaccinations and Injections* (Oldsmar, Florida: Natural Hygiene Press, 1985)

Chaitow, L., *Vaccination and Immunization: Dangers, Delusions and Alternatives* (Saffron Walden, England: C.W. Daniel, 1987)

Coulter, H.L., and Fisher, B.L. *DPT- A Shot in the Dark* (New York: Avery Publishing Group, 1987)

Head, C.J., *An Educated Decision*, (Lavender Hill Homœopathic Centre, London SW11 1PJ, 1995)

James, W., *Immunisation:The Reality Behind the Myth* (USA: Bergin and Garvey Inc., 1988)

Moskowitz, R., *The Case Against Immunisations* (photocopy of article available from The Society of Homœopaths, 2 Artizan Road, Northampton NN1 4HU, 1983)

Neustaedter, R., *The Immunisation Decision: A Guide for Parents* (California: North Atlantic Books, 1990)

Phillips, A., *Dispelling Vaccination Myths*, (York, England: Prometheus, 1999) available from Helios Pharmacy

Scheibner, V., *Vaccination: The Medical Assault on the Immune System*, (178 Goretts Leap Rd, NSW 2785, Australia: Scheibner, 1993)

UK Department of Health, *Immunisation Against Infectious Disease* (HMSO Publications, 1990)

What Doctors Don't Tell You, *The Vaccination Bible,* (WDDTY, 1991)

HOMŒOPATHY

Castro, M., *The Complete Homœopathy Handbook* (London: Macmillan, 1990)

Cummings, S., & Ullman, D., *Everybody's Guide to Homœopathic Medicines* (London: Gollancz, 1984)

Lessell, C.B, *The World Travellers' Manual of Homœopathy* (Saffron Walden, England: C.W.Daniel, 1993)

Lockie, Dr. A., *The Family Guide to Homœopathy* (London: Hamish Hamilton, 1989)

Phatak, S., *Materia Medica of Homœopathic Medicines* (Delhi, India: IBPS, 1977)

Speight, P., *Before Calling the Doctor* (Saffron Walden, England: C.W.Daniel, 1976)

HERBS

Bartram, T., *Encyclopedia of Herbal Medicine*, (Christchurch, Dorset, England: Grace, 1995)

Grieve, M., *A Modern Herbal* (London: Penguin, 1931)

Hoffman, D., *The Holistic Herbal* (Shaftesbury, Dorset: Element, 1983)

Tierra, M., *The Way of Herbs* (Santa Cruz, USA: Orenda /United Press, 1980)

ESSENTIAL OILS

Curtis, S., *Essential Oils*, (London: Aurum, 1996)

Davis, P., *Aromatherapy: An A-Z* (Saffron Walden, England: C.W.Daniel, 1988)

Tisserand, R., *The A-Z of Aromatherapy* (Saffron Walden, England: C.W.Daniel, 1980)

Valnet, J., *The Practice of Aromatherapy* (Saffron Walden, England: C.W.Daniel, 1980)

INDEX